SPLAT!

An Introduction to
Sploshing
&
Food Play

Wamlanta

Copyright © 2018 Wamlanta

All rights reserved.

ISBN: 9781729188309

Dedicated to all three Stooges.

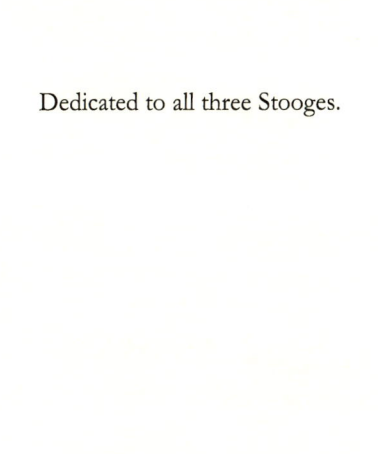

CONTENTS

	Prologue	i
1	You're Into What	8
2	Be Prepared: Equipment	14
3	Foodstuffs	20
4	Non-Foodstuffs	26
5	You're Not Alone: Real Stories	28
6	Bound to be Pied	40
7	Additional Resources	42
8	Taking the Plunge	44

PROLOGUE

"We had a bet," the attendant said as she loaded the last of fifty five tubs of Cool Whip into my car. "what's all this for?"

My heart raced as I suddenly realized I should have taken a few moments to prepare a small lie before picking up this massive order. In fact, I paid extra for the personal shopper service to avoid any sort of confrontation. After all, who wants to explain being caught in Kroger with a buggy full of cool whip? Of course I'd already purchased the tins, tarps, and other essentials for what was going to be an interesting evening. But that didn't change the fact that a stranger, a fairly attractive stranger at that, was asking me about my carload of non-dairy whipped topping. "It's for a charity event," I shamelessly lied. "A women's health charity; it's for a bunch of pies in the face". A half-truth. Maybe three-quarters, since it had nothing to do with charity. Or health, for that matter. 'Oh, please don't ask which charity.'

She smiled, "Oh, that's cool. Most people thought it was for some sort of youth event. You're not going to get pied, are you?"

"Actually, yes." I said confidently. "They're all for me." That part was true. However the full truth doesn't include a women's health event but rather a room full of leather-clad femme dommes at the local dungeon. Somehow I think sharing the whole truth might have been a bit more awkward. Maybe next time I'll come clean if the Kroger is far enough away from home.

Heh, clean.

Later in the day I managed to bring all but 10 tubs up to the hotel room, along with a well-stocked kit that included all the tins, towels, and tools I needed to create a successful evening. Sitting at the desk at the Tucker Doubletree, I spent the next couple of hours listening to the television and filling massive ziplock bags with thawed out cool whip, which isn't as easy as one might expect. My plan included using different colors in an effort to keep it visually interesting, so I mixed a good amount of food coloring into each bag. Fortunately it worked perfectly and I ended up with 8 large bags full of cool whip, nearly all dyed in green, blue, and purple fluorescent colors.

The shower at 1763, the local dungeon, is larger than my entire bathroom, and is perfect for this sort of thing. By the time everything was prepared, the walls and floor were covered in plastic, tins were laid out, (some of the already filled), and the assistants knew what to do. I got cheeky with the blue painter's tape and taped two large arrows pointing to the center, where I would spend the next hour or so being a target for these awesome people. Word spread quickly that we were about to begin, and suddenly a line of dommes stood in line with one purpose, and that was to throw a pie in my face. Or at least my general direction, depending on their aim.

1

YOU'RE INTO WHAT?

Are you reading a fetish book in public? You naughty bastard.

There's an unfortunate perception that if you get off on something other than the most basic act of sexual congress then you are a pervert or deviant. It's an unfair accusation, especially when statistics reveal that the overwhelming majority of individuals have at least one kink or fetish. In a recent UK survey of 2,300 people, 75 percent report having at least one fetish while over a quarter of respondents enjoy more than one. Even so, pearls are clutched when it is discovered friends, neighbors, or family members find feet sexually arousing. It's shocking when we learn that the most boring of people enjoy worshiping their domme or being a "Daddy" to a 30 year old Little. To paraphrase Heath Ledger's Joker: "If, tomorrow night, I bring a can of whipped cream into the bedroom for some risqué fun, nobody panics. But when I inflate one little pool and fill it up with cool whip, everyone loses their minds!" These needlessly closed-minded opinions result in shame and embarrassment for too many people. But that does not stop a single hypocrite from secretly donning a shiny leather mask to become the

Phantom Ass Slapper while cloistered away in their own bedroom.[1] Rather than dwelling on negatives and critics, we are going to focus on the positives, namely exploring a new and unique fetish you can incorporate in your life. Perhaps you've dipped a toe into getting messy. After all, who hasn't licked a dollop of cream off their partner's nipples? Or perhaps drizzled a bit of chocolate syrup on their partner's cock only to seductively lick it off. Sploshing is like that, except a ridiculous amount more.

What is Sploshing?

The term sploshing came about as a result of a now defunct UK fetish magazine named Splosh!. While the UK was sploshing about, so to speak, Americans adopted the label of WAM, or "wet and messy". These terms, splosh/sploshing/splosher are interchangeable with WAM/wamming/wammer. However, in this book we will mostly use the terms derived from splosh, though don't feel compelled to use one over the other; use whichever one feels right to you. (Personally I use the term "sploshing" with someone new to the fetish, and "wamming" with someone familiar with the community. No clue why, it just happens that way.) There are a few other words you'll likely learn later, but let's start with these for now.

Sploshing is the erotic act of wet and messy play where participants start out clean and end up a dirty, filthy mess. This can be accomplished with a variety of substances, ranging from all manner of sweet or savory food, mud, certain chemicals, or just plain old water. This isn't as cut and dry as something like pegging, for instance, where your partner is ether wearing a strap-on and penetrating your ass or she is not. In this fetish there is a

---

[1] No ass is safe

lot of wiggle room in what constitutes sploshing. You can use a little or a lot, wear clothes or cover your birthday suit in birthday cake. You could do it on a bed, sitting in a shower, under a bucket, or in the middle of a bog. It's up to you, and it's quite versatile when paired with other fetishes. Getting messy is a delight for the senses, teasing your sight, hearing, taste, smell, and touch, all at the same time. It's the sight of your partner covered in boldly-colored goo that drips off his body. Or the sensation of being helplessly engulfed by a barrage of whipped cream as she sandwiches two pies on your head. Perhaps for you it's the sound of sinking deeper into a cool mud pit on a hot day. In many ways it's too broad a term, but here we are, attempting to explore the root of what sploshing is. As your adventure begins you may find one or two things that tickles your fancy, which is great. But to avoid confusion in the future it helps to know what sploshing generally doesn't cover before we continue forward. Note that this list is neither exhaustive nor is it intended critical or judgmental. I fully support you enjoying these activities, they just don't happen to be sploshing.

1. **Sploshing is not bodily fluids**, including feces, urine, vomit, semen, or any other possible substance that is produced by the human body. As an example, while a lot of watersports includes wetting pants and panties, it is generally not welcome under the WAM umbrella. That's not to say you cannot enjoy both watersports and sploshing, it is however considered a separate fetish. So if your partner reveals to you they're a splosher, the last thing you should expect is being peed on (or insert bodily function of your choice). But don't let the rigidity of the definition of sploshing stop you from doing what you want. You're an adult, dammit. If you want to go down the golden river, take that trip, just don't forget your towel.

2. **Sploshing is not using vegetables as dildos**. Perhaps looking seductive while shopping for produce is a

good way to communicate your desires to your fellow shoppers, but it certainly doesn't encourage any wet and messy activity. The presence of food does not make it a sploshing activity.

3. **Sploshing is not using a bit of whip cream and chocolate to spice up the bedroom.** Now, don't get me wrong, this can be a blast, and I highly recommend it if you haven't tried it in so far. In fact, while squirting cream and chocolate over your partner and licking it off isn't in and of itself sploshing, can very well be considered gateway activity, (something we'll cover more in depth in a later chapter). It's a great way to introduce sploshing to your partner, and it's likely the most common way people non-fetishists get messy in the bedroom. If after you've read this book nothing changes, perhaps you'll be tempted to squeeze that syrup bottle a little harder, or better yet take the cap off completely.

Why Sploshing?

Obviously this is one of the stranger fetishes, because who comes up with the idea that smearing food all over their partner is fun? Well, at the scale we are talking about it's not common, but the principle of enjoying getting messy isn't anything new. Why was 9 ½ Weeks so erotic? Why do we like mud wrestling? Or better yet, why did the WWE have pudding matches in above ground pools filled with pudding and whipped cream? We have always looked at getting messy as erotic and seductive, but we have also looked at it in very lighthearted ways. It just so happens in those innocent, "vanilla" instances of getting messy that many messy fetishists were born. Of course everyone is different and has their own story. For some it might have started with watching people get pied or slimed on a television show. 80's and early 90's kids in the US and Canada will remember You Can't Do That on Television, the Canadian kids television show broadcast on

Nickelodeon. In fact, even 30 years later, every drop of green slime Nickelodeon pours can thank YCDTOTV for inspiration. At the same time, across the pond, UK viewers would have watched shows such as Tiswas, Get Your Own Back, or Noel's House Party, all of which included being pied, dropped into a vat of gunge (slime) or being sat in a booth and deluged by a wave of gunge from above. At some point in our youth, our perverted brains see this and a subconscious switch is flipped.[2] This isn't a technical book, so if you want to read further on the development of human sexuality and fetishes, feel free. Anecdotally, in the same way it's awkward when nudity pops up on TV when your parents are in the room, I recall being embarrassed when someone was slimed. I didn't realize it back then, but hindsight can reveal lots of things.

Who Should Read This Book

Since this is neither technical or philosophical, you shouldn't feel overwhelmed. Rather, this is an introduction to practical sploshing, a guide you can use either by yourself or with a partner to introduce wet and messy play into your repertoire. Here you'll find tips and tricks to make your messy fun safe and easy to clean up. You may also want to use this book as a way to introduce sploshing to your partner. I sincerely hope you do so, and in fact, that is one of the primary reasons for writing this book. Obviously everyone is going to have a different degree of comfort when it comes to communicating their hidden fetishes. It takes revealing a side you may have never shared with anyone, and that can be scary. But communication is important, and understanding that your desires are neither wrong nor shameful is paramount. Is there a possibility your partner may not be accepting of

---

[2] I'm not a mental health professional; this is just my perspective.

your fetish? Of course. And hopefully they won't shame you for having these desires. (If they do make you feel ashamed and humiliated for your desires, you've learned a bit about who your partner is.) But if you never share who you are, you'll never be whole; if you never express your hidden desires, they may never be fulfilled. Life is too short to ignore who you really are.

To the men and women whose partner gave them this book, I ask that you read this with an open mind. Know that they've trusted you with their very private secret. If they've taken the step of opening up to you about their fetish, they're probably, at this moment, more vulnerable than they've ever been. I know this puts you in a weird position, and I hope you accept this responsibility with a kind and graceful heart. Don't misunderstand, our purpose is not to guilt you into doing something with which you are uncomfortable; I'm not saying you should appease their fetish if you're repulsed by it. No means no, and everyone has the right to choose whether or not to acquiesce their partner's desires. But there's a huge difference between saying "I really don't want to do that; it's not for me" and "you freak, absolutely not!". Be kind. But if you make the choice to take a few squishy steps into your partner's world, I hope you approach sploshing with a willingness to dive in, be silly, and share in a sensual and erotic fetish your partner loves.

2

BE PREPARED - EQUIPMENT

Like anything worthwhile, sploshing is not something you can approach haphazardly. It requires strategy to plan for what is going to be an absolutely awesome day. Generally speaking your day is going to be split into three distinct phases: prep, play, and cleanup. And since the size of your messy session dictates your prep and cleanup strategy, we will look at small, medium, and large scale play sessions so you can have an idea of what it takes to put these together. While it is impractical to detail the endless number of ingredients you can play with, we will look at a large variety so you can be well prepared as you try new things.

Equipment

Sploshing indoors is going to have some challenges, and every step along the way is really dictated by your play space. Not every home has a room-sized shower, complete with a hose powerful enough to clean everyone and everything. You have to consider protecting the furniture, floors, and walls of your house, along with making the area safe in the event of an emergency. It is always good, no matter what size session you are organizing, to have both a wet and dry towel handy so you can quickly clean off your face and eyes.

Small and Solo Sessions

For a small session, and this is especially good for solo sploshers, the tub is the perfect spot for something like a pie or two, or a bucket of gunge. The challenge here is, where does the mess go when you're done? If you're using pie with shells or even a cake, you can't simply shove everything down the drain. Anything more than a small amount of solids leads to having a very awkward conversation with your local plumber. Instead, line your tub with 2mm plastic drop cloth sheeting which you can wrap up and easily dispose of in a plastic garbage bag. This keeps your mess contained, and you can clean yourself off rather quickly since you're already in the tub. A hair catcher in the tub is perfect for preventing any large chunks from making their way down the drain, so you can wash off without worrying about your plumbing.

Certain types of gunge/slime are perfect for the tub and can be washed down the drain without any problems. As such they do not require the plastic drop cloth or any excessive measures, though this is not the case with all options. Look to a later chapter for which types of gunge are drain safe, and which require a little more effort to dispose.

Medium Sessions

So you've gotten a taste for getting messy and you want to make it a little more fun? Time to move out of the bathroom and into an area more spacious. Two places will work perfectly: in the bedroom (and on the bed if yours is large enough) and in the living room. Regardless of which you choose, ensure you have a path of plastic or towels leading to the bathroom. Hide the good towels (so you don't accidentally leave an eternal chocolate impression of your face and hands), and set out some you can afford to lose, or at least keep hidden from guests. Note that when you finally make it into the shower, certain items you use might make for a dangerously slippery situation. Line the tub with a towel to give you a safe place to stand. Experience will let you know when you need this, but this is a safe bet for your first few times.

The easier of the two is going to be the living room. If you're like most people you have a couch, a couple of tables, a chair, and a television. Push back everything you can to make room, and lay tarps down on the ground and any furniture you plan on keeping clean. This is a basic setup, and thinner sheeting can be used for anywhere you're not going to be standing, so covering the walls and furniture with 1.5 or 2mm thick plastic is sufficient. Thicker, 2.5mm sheeting, is generally used where you play to prevent punching a hole through the plastic. All of these drop cloths can be secured to each other, the walls, and furniture with painter's tape. I recommend a wider roll of tape, at least 2", in order to keep the sheets from slipping free. It might run you $6 a roll, but it will last a long time if you don't try to tape every inch of the room.

If you choose to adapt this to the bedroom, the larger the bed the better. There are a couple of ways to setup the room. As always, use plastic drop cloths to cover sensitive areas in the room. If you want to play on the bed you can do one of a few things. You can remove the pillows and cover the mattress with plastic sheeting. If you choose this option, be sure to tuck the sheeting in and tape it, to ensure it doesn't creep up and expose your linens. Or you could have a fitted sheet for just this occasion where you protect the mattress with plastic, and place a fitted sheet over top. Alternatively, rubber sheets are effective, though much more expensive and less disposable. (For this you have you balance whether you are willing to go through the cleaning process, or if it would be easier to simply fold everything in and throw it away). These are some of the more comfortable ways to set up your bedroom since you're playing on fabric and not on plastic. Note that it's a good idea to also place plastic on the floor around the bed, along with having a trail of plastic leading to the bathroom. That cheap $2 plastic sheet can mean the difference between renting a carpet cleaner or not. I prefer not.

These are great setups for pies and various foodstuffs, but not for an overly excessive amount of pourable mess. You can get away with a couple of gallons, but remember you will have to dispose of everything somehow. Which leads us to . . .

Large Sessions

Are you expecting company today? Not anymore. This is where it can get a little crazy, a little more difficult to set up and clean, but it is absolutely one of the most amazing and fun things you'll ever experience. This works best with a larger room and an open floor, and you might need to move some furniture out of the way. The basics still apply. Plastic sheeting on the walls and floor, a path to the bathroom, towels to clean your face and eyes. If you've done a medium session or two, you have this down pat. Now it's time to inflate the pool.

Yes, you heard that right.

There are a couple of different kinds I would recommend. The first would be a small round pool. If your sploshing is one sided where only one person is getting messy, this isn't a bad option. One can sit in the middle or on a seat. But if this is more of a couples activity, I recommend the Intex Swim Center Family Inflatable Pool. Measuring 120" x 72" x 22", this is perfect for all manner of frolicking. Make no mistake, this is a big pool. It's going to take up a large amount of floor space, so if it'll fit, go for it. You might need something a bit smaller, which is fine; any of them will work. I like the larger sizes since the materials are a bit thicker, will last longer, and the walls of the pool are much more sturdy. Do yourself a favor and acquire a pump that will both inflate and deflate since you're going to reuse this. This is possible because rather than explaining to the neighbors why you're hosing down a chocolate covered pool, you're simply going to line the pool with another drop cloth. I recommend 2.5mm , and the largest size you can find to ensure the edges aren't pulled into the mess. Your goal is to minimize spillage as you wrap up and dispose of everything when you're done. If you're using a lot of thick gunge and slime you might have to dispose of some of it before wrapping up the plastic. This can be accomplished a couple of different ways.

If you're putting a session together this large, chances are you're using pretty big buckets full of all kinds of fun things. Chances are most of the ingredients you're using can be disposed of in either the garbage disposal or toilet. The latter feels risky, but I have never had an issue with it. Alternatively you can use a garbage disposal. Just be careful and take your time. Start out by refilling the buckets with the gunge in the bottom of the pool. Maybe it's cake batter, oatmeal, or natrosol, or a fun combination of the three. Pull the plastic back to force the goo onto one side of the pool. WIth a small pitcher, begin to scoop the gunge back into the larger buckets. These can be transported to the bathroom or kitchen. If flushing, pour into the bowl slowly while it is flushing. It might take a few times, but it's ok. Just be patient. If using the garbage disposal, run the water while you pour into an already running disposal. Once you feel there is a manageable amount of mess left in the pool, start to pull the plastic up until you are holding all the edges. If you do this correctly, there should be a ball of goo trapped behind some clear plastic. Carefully place this into a 55 gallon plastic bag. Now I should stop you and say, yes, I buy cheap plastic drop cloths. I buy the cheapest ones I can, because they do the job. In the name of everything that is good and clean, don't cheap out on your garbage bags. There's about 1.5mm difference between success and chaos, and the last thing you want is your neighbor wondering if you just birthed an alien baby after your play session rips through the world's cheapest garbage bag and spills out on your front lawn. Do. Not Be. Cheap.

No matter what size of a session you're planning, having a plan is essential and will make it a much more enjoyable experience. Never neglect the basics, and always consider safety.

3

FOODSTUFFS

Foodstuffs are generally sorted into two different categories: sweet and savory. Everyone has their own preference when it comes to what they enjoy getting messy with. I've noticed a very strong correlation between savory and humiliation, though that isn't always the case. I personally prefer sweet over savory with oatmeal really being the only non-sweet foodstuff I enjoy. To each their own. If you prefer gravy over custard and that makes you happy, have at it! Really anything you can think of can be used for sploshing, but we'll go through a few examples to give you ideas.

Sweet

Whipped Cream

This is the original, most basic thing you can use. It tastes and feels wonderful, but there are some things to consider. Whipped cream is a dairy product, and so as it melts or sits on your skin, it might produce an off-putting smell as your body heat slowly sours the cream. Real whip cream is very fun, but using an oil based product such as Cool Whip will minimize any sort of smell on your body after the fact. In addition, Cool Whip does not melt in the way whip cream disintegrates into liquid. It's much more stable, and you can sufficiently prep without worrying about your pies melting.

Chocolate/Pancake/Golden Syrup

We might as well get all the basics out of the way. Chocolate syrup is easy, fun, delicious, and messy. One of the biggest "vanilla" complaints about getting messy is they "don't like to get sticky". And they use the past experience of a lover using something like chocolate syrup, who maybe smeared it around their body made them into an uncomfortable, sticky, mess. Well, when you use a small amount and smear it on the skin, and this applies for most of these items, when you use a small amount it's going to dry out very quickly, leaving nothing but sticky skin and an unfortunate experience. Rather, if you use a whole bottle, especially in conjunction with other foods, it's not going to dry out. Rather than sticky, you're going to be gooey, slippery, and chocolaty.

Pancake and golden syrups are going to be a little different. Most pancake syrup is corn syrup based and is thinner in consistency than most Chocolate, while golden syrup is much thicker. Since it is much thinner, pancake syrup has a tendency to dry out quicker than chocolate, so be aware of that possibility. Golden syrup is thicker, heavier, and pours slower. It's generally more expensive, so you're probably not going to get five gallons worth. But it has its place and some people really enjoy the weight and sensation of a jar of it being poured all over them. You won't know unless you try, right?

Cake Batter & Oatmeal

These are some of my favorite ingredients, and their function is similar, so we'll merge them together.

Cake batter and oatmeal are some of the best ways to create buckets of slime/gunge at home. They're fairly viscous so they're going to retain heat. You can dye them any color you like to add an extra dimension of fun to your session. Want to be covered in green slime just like on TV? Now you can!

For cake batter I recommend store bought white cake mix. Of course you can use chocolate if you like, but if you're dying it you'll want the most neutral color possible. White is perfect and takes on colors really well. Some people prefer to add oil and eggs just like they're making a real cake. You can definitely do this, though I just use warm water and mix by hand to the consistency I enjoy. It takes a little trial and error, and you can do it differently. But remember you can't take water away. If you make it too thin, that's what it is. Additionally, you can also use a hand mixer, immersion blender, or even a mixing attachment for your electric drill if you are mixing a large amount.

Oatmeal is very similar in that you simply pour quick oats into a bucket and add water, but be aware that if you let it sit too long, it's going to thicken up. That's not necessarily a bad thing, but it's a little more forgiving in that regard. If you initially add too much water the oats should absorb most of it, bringing it back to a more friendly consistency. Warmer water is great as the thickness of the oatmeal will retain the heat for much longer. I like leaving it for one of the last items in a play session as the temperature is still good, making it feel like a warm, gooey blanket cascading over your body. It has such an incredible weight, and the sensation is unlike anything you've experienced.

If you're dying either cake batter or oatmeal, you'll probably use much more food coloring than you expect to.

It's fine; it won't stain your skin after being diluted in your bucket of slime, but concentrated it absolutely will. So unless you want to look like you spent your weekend strangling a Smurf, be careful.

Pies

To put it simply, pies are awesome. There are so many different flavors, textures, styles, and techniques. The most basic pie you could make is a can of squirt cream on a paper plate. This the most budget, quick thing you could use as a pie. If you really want to use that, enjoy it. Personally I'll leave that to the people who lost workplace bets, so let's see what we can do to improve it one step at at time.

Tins - Real tins can make a lot of difference. They're larger, hold more ingredients, and carry enough weight to be thrown. While this can get expensive, it's not too bad when you stock up during sales.

Crusts - Ah, real crusts. Now this requires a bit more effort. There are pre-made graham cracker crusts, but I find these make things a bit too scratchy afterwards. A great alternative is a frozen crust already in the tin which you can bake ahead of time. You can leave the crust in the tin, or if you're extra skilled, remove the pie from the tin so you're just smushing or throwing a completely intact pie. If you leave it in the tin, it's helpful to crimp the pie in your hand, squeezing it to break up the crust so it releases from the tin when you pie your partner (or self).

Fillings - Pies can be filled with any number of items, including fruit compote and fillings, puddings, and custard. Chocolate and vanilla pudding is an easy one to use. Both will give some contrast to the topping, and will give you a different taste. Note many fruit filling such as cherry and blueberry may stain your skin. So use these with caution.

Toppings - The basic pie topping as I mentioned, is the squirt cream. Now if you've gone to the trouble of making an awesome pie, you're not going to want to top it with something that's going to melt and make you sad, do you? Of course not. One upgrade is cool whip. It won't melt, it feels great, and will not make your skin smell in the same way a dairy based whipped cream will. A step above that is buttercream frosting. Usually one of the warehouse clubs, such as Costco or Sam's Club, will sell 5 pound buckets of buttercream frosting. While I have never used this option, others swear by it, and will fill their pies with just buttercream. Experiment and find out what is right for you.

Frozen - Your grocer should have a few frozen pie options in their freezer. I've never been impressed by their offerings, but some people really enjoy them. If you are lucky enough to have a Gordon's Food Service (GFS) store nearby, they sell frozen pies that have been used by multiple producers. They're larger than those in the grocery store as they are commercial quality and size. I highly recommend these if you want something simple.

Bakery-made - This is by far the most expensive option, and can lead to some weird looks if you buy a lot of them, but the quality really cannot be beat. These are usually large, filled, and heavy. Most any bakery can make them. The downside is you'll have to personally order them, so if you can overcome that and have money to burn, this might be the best option for you.

Savory

I have zero experience in savory options, but I can say from observation, savory tends to be well adopted in the humiliation aspect of WAM, though that's not always the case. Some are simply more focused on textures and how various substances are applied. Items like ketchup, mayonnaise, beans, spaghetti, and gravy are certainly suitable items to use, and many people enjoy using them either alone or alongside sweet stuffs. You will definitely experience a unique sensation when a cold tin of Spaghetti O's are dumped into your unmentionables. Be careful with edges, though. Safety first.

4

NON-FOODSTUFFS

There are many messy options that don't include raiding your pantry. Some are natural while some are not. This doesn't mean they're dangerous, however, each of these will require a certain level of care and preparation above and beyond your typical messy session. The goal is to remain safe, secure, and without injury, while still having fun.

Gunge - Gunge is a general term. If you're watching scenes from UK programs such as Get Your Own Back, or Nickelodeon slime from anywhere in the world, what you're seeing, in general terms, is an industrial thickener, often food grade. Some of the items used include Natrosol, Metholcelluose, Guar Gum, and Xanthian Gum. While the latter two can be found in any health food store, the former are more difficult to come by. All of these are available online through various retailers and come with complete instructions. You may even want to construct a gunge tank to make it easier to dump on your lover/victim/self. Since these items are thickeners, they can be thick and chunky or very thin. They can be very slippery (Natrosol is every bit slippery as lube), so be very careful when using these. It might be helpful to have a wet towel to stand or kneel on if someone is pouring these over you. This will keep you from slipping around.

Mud - I don't have a lot of experience playing in the mud, so if your desire is to get muddy, I would recommend researching local options before taking my advice. If you experience this out in nature you'll have to deal with, well, nature. Bugs, snakes, and hikers exist out in the wilderness, so be aware of your surrounding, and don't die. Some choose to construct their own mud and clay pits at home, often supplied by online retailers who sell kaolin clay by the boxful. Note this is not extremely easy to dispose of. You don't want to pour mud down the drain, so be aware of that before you fill a pool with your favorite silky clay.

Shaving foam - If you've ever seen a clown hit by a pie, chances are it was a shaving cream pie, or one made out of soap). These are super easy to make, extremely inexpensive, and fun. The downside is incorporating other sexual activities is more difficult. Because who wants the taste of soap or shaving cream in their mouth? That doesn't mean you can't have some quick fun and wash off before jumping in bed. Just don't slip.

J Lube - This is a unique product found on Amazon that can bring a lot of fun times into your life. Each 10oz bottle will make 6-8 gallons of lube. Yes, you heard that right. Less water makes it thicker, and regular table salt breaks it down, so it's easy to dispose of. It's non-toxic and shouldn't irritate the skin. For $30 you can have 10 gallons of thick, fun slime to play around with.

5

YOU'RE NOT ALONE - REAL STORIES

One unique aspect of the Wet and Messy world is there is an actual online community that has been around for over 20 years. www.umd.net (The Ultimate Messy Directory) is an online forum and general portal for all things wet and messy. Today you'll find hundreds of producers putting out over a thousand messy videos every year. But in the beginning, much of the discussion included finding scenes in movies and tv shows. Entrepreneurial perverts would compile cliptapes to sell, though a few producers sold what people really wanted to see. Namely attractive models getting wet, messy, and muddy.

Leah

Leah, AKA Messygirl, was one of the earliest producers in the WAM community. She was gracious enough to answer a few questions regarding her experience in the community and as a splosher.

Please tell me a little about yourself and how long have you been into and how did you first discover WAM?

My name is Leah. I'm a Midwest girl and I'm 53. My first experience with WAM was at age 12. I recall walking barefoot in mud and the sensation and wet sound triggered something in me. I wanted to feel it all over my body.

There's playing around, and then there's that first real messy session. Describe your first real messy session. Not just what you used and who you were with, but other things as well. Anticipation, perhaps? How long did you plan? Was there a risk of getting caught?

When I was old enough to stay home alone at age 13, I would use this time to experience total mud play in the backyard. I was fortunate to have a private location in the backyard to experience this. Basically, I would dig my own private mud pit and play in it. I started out in a swimsuit and would always end up nude. I discovered masturbation with an orgasm doing this. There was a risk of getting caught, but the sensation of it all just was too strong to resist doing it. I then started to experience other messy things inside. I would actually let a bowl of ice cream melt and pour it over my head in the bathtub. I also used my dads shaving cream to make pies. I used a wash rag hold it all. I would pie my face and then rub it all over my body. I watch myself in the mirror when I did this. I had no idea why I liked doing this, but knew I had to do it and it would always end with me masturbating.

Do you consider WAM, at least as you incorporate it in your life, to be a sexual act? Would you consider this to be a genuine fetish for you? Does your partner share that fetish?

Yes, WAM is very sexual with me and even though my partner is not a true wammer, he does enjoy watching me reveal in my fetish.

How did you go about introducing your partner to WAM? Did he take some coaxing; what was his reaction?

Well, I got to know him first. Once I found out he

was open minded, I told him.

How often do you incorporate WAM into your personal life?

I will incorporate wam and sex with my partner. It really is the only time I WAM now. Solo WAM is no longer needed, since I have a partner to enjoy it with. So when we fuck he will pie me or dunk my head in a bucket of batter. My strongest orgasms happen when I combined WAM with sex. Much of what you seen in our Messygirl blowjob shoots has happened to me in my personal sex life.

One interesting thing about WAM is the internet community that started over 20 years ago. Do you feel encouraged by the community at large, or are you indifferent? Or, how much would you say the community contributes to your identity as a wammer?

Well, WAM has become a huge business and I know for a fact many of the so called wam models only do it for the money. I came into this to express my love of the fetish and it then grew into a business. I never thought it would become this, but glad we can still express our true love of WAM in this way.

What advice would you give a person introducing wam to their partner?

Make WAM about the both of you, not just about yourself. As long as they are enjoying it with you, it's all good.

◆◆◆

There are lots of individuals and couples who share their messy exploits on the internet, but in my opinion very few can hold a candle to Anthony and Suzette. It's a story of mutual respect and openness that can only strenghten a relationship. They were gracious enough to share a little bit about their journey.

Anthony and Suzette

Which one brought WAM to the table?

(Anthony) I did.

How did you introduce your fetish into the relationship?

(A) Over time. I did not bring it up at all as a thing until three years in. But along the way I hinted at the idea. I would ask to add cream or chocolate to love making, (you know, the vanilla stuff that most people do), to gauge were she was at with that. She took to it fine and I pushed the threshold here and there. Finally, one day she found a WAM video on my PC and she asked me about it and I came clean (no PUN) and explained what I liked. She asked to see some content that I enjoy most. She said that looks like fun and general was supportive.

To Suzette, what were your initial thoughts and concerns, if any? How were they overcome?

(Suzette) Sure, why did he keep this hidden for so long? I now have the cheat code to unlock his inner most desires and that's just plain fun to have! Being an outsider to the WAM world I had no idea how things worked. Anthony likes stuff poured into his clothing and generally enjoys goopy food items. He likes cakes, puddings, or batter, things of that such. Seemed like a large waste of food, a lot a prep and break down, and costly at the end of the day. It makes him happy, so I can get by that. I also had to learn what makes a messy girl sexy exactly? Take your expectations of looking pretty and clean as a girl and then flip that over knowing he just wants to throw you in the mud. Kinda interesting world view to digest.

To Anthony, when did you first discover WAM? Did you find it on your own or did someone introduce it to you? What pushed you over the edge to get messy for the first time?

(A) I always knew I liked WAM. I don't remember ever not thinking WAM thoughts when thinking erotically.

I guess what made me try it for the first time was thinking how naughty it would be to do. That feeling of doing something wrong and it feeling so right. I think every session I have now chases that feeling but has never came close. Don't get me wrong... it's still bliss! but nothing like that first time.

There's playing around, and then there's that first real messy session. Describe your first real messy session as a couple.

(S) We have it on video! It used to be in the UMD store though it was not put up till years after we first did it. We opened a small store with 5-6 videos and that was added as one. I wanted to make him a video like the ones he showed me and just be a big tease. I thought it was fun. By that time, we talked about it a fair bit and I had a good idea what to do. We planned the dress and the materials to be things he enjoyed most.

(A) I don't think I'd change a thing. At that time, it was the most amazing thing that ever happened to me. I'm so lucky to have her.

Do you consider WAM, at least as you incorporate it in your life, to be a sexual act? Would you consider this to be a genuine fetish for you? To the newcomer, would you say you have personally adopted this as a fetish or is it something you're doing to appease your partner?

(A) Yes full blown fetish. WAM IS MY SEX LIFE. I need it to get off at this point. If I'm watching porn its WAM... nothing else does it for me... Sure we have sex... and I get off... but nothing brings to the end like WAM does.

(S) I do it to appease him. I don't think I'd never do it with another partner god forbid we got divorced. That's not to say it don't enjoy it. Getting him off and sex wild makes me sex wild. Some of my best orgasms have been covered in goop. So, I'm not sure how that classifies exactly.

How often do you incorporate WAM into your personal life?

(A) We have what we call a "session" at least once a month. These are planned out. We sometimes will see things on sale and if the prices are really good we'll get what we need and go for it. "That's a POPUP session" In the winter months when it's cold here that number drops to zero though. We both don't enjoy getting covered in things when it's cold.

One interesting thing about WAM is the internet community that started over 20 years ago. Like myself you're not very active or vocal on the site, so I'm guessing the majority of your engagement is passive. Do you feel encouraged by the community at large, or are you indifferent? Or, how much would you say the wider community contributes to your identity as a wammer?

(A) So we closed our store down a long time ago because of taxes. UMD needed us to fill out tax paper to get paid and we have a family guy who does our taxes. Him seeing "loverbuns INC" with 300 bucks in taxable income would be questionable at best. We originally made the store to just get money to WAM with. 100% of what we made went back into WAM sessions. We never filmed videos that people where asking for. I made the content I liked to see, and if you wanted to buy it... great! If not, no skin off my back. That being said, after the store closed a year or so later Sue said wouldn't it be fun to just throw all the videos out there for free for the UMD. We did it one by one. We planned to do one a week and that did not go well. You can look at the last few posts on my old account "MESSYANT". The bottom line was no one cared at the time. For two video releases we barely got any thanks or acknowledgment. I'll be honest, I felt slighted by that. Thousands of thread views and video views and like four people saying something. At the time someone would post a random pic of their wife with a little yogurt on her boobs and the forums would explode. Here I am giving away free intimate videos of our sex lives and I got 4 replies. Maybe its was my ego or something but was a blow to me. Sue and I spoke, and she said fuck it... Why do this if no one is giving any feedback? After all we thought that was the most fun part of the whole thing. Especially her as she enjoy hearing compliments about how she looked. I enjoyed seeing people taking to my work, that's what motivated me to film and then give it away. So we both came to a decision to not give the rest away. I closed that account and left for about a year or two I think. At some point I made this account Now I lurk and drop a snarky comment once and a while. The video on my profile was a gift to a friend on the forum. Yes its public but I really wanted to share it with one guy.

What advice would you give to a person introducing WAM to their partner?

(S) Easy just be straight forward and explain what you like. Yes I understand that hearing those words come out of your mouth to another is going to be weird but think about the person the other end. You cant expect me to understand all the complexity of what your asking for just by saying "I like to get messy". If you really want to please your partner and care about what they want it should be a no brainer. Have a long talk and tell me all the history of the fetish and why it makes you tic. Me understanding where my husband was coming from really made me understand why this was important to him. Sure he could do it without me if he wanted to, but the fact that he is willing to open up and share that part of himself with me brings us closer together.

◆◆◆

When I started looking for people to interview, Leah was the first person to come to mind, primarily because I knew from her posts on The Ultimate Messy Directory that she was a real wammer, someone who truly enjoys it and isn't in it just for the money. Because she's right, many of the models only do this to get paid. There's nothing wrong with doing that, of course. But this purpose of this book is more on incorporating sploshing into your personal life, as opposed to becoming a model. Because the world is saturated with good intentioned folks just getting messy for money, it makes finding the right person to interview that much more difficult. I wanted to find the right people on my own, not just through a forum request, so I browsed profiles on UMD for any indication of people who are actually into WAM. Then I ran across a blog written by MyPieRogative.

Also an American, Ms. MyPieRogative was very gracious in allowing me to reprint her first experience. What makes this narrative so great is it's from the perspective of someone who had WAM introduced to them. The awkward conversation, the anticipation leading up to that first time, it's all there. And, as promised, if this makes the NYT Bestsellers list, I'll send $20.00 your way.

MyPieRogative
My First Pie

We laid in bed in my messy tiny efficiency apartment. All cuddled up after after love making. I asked him what his "thing" is. "Everyone has something" I said. He looked nervous and smirked. I was very curious at this point! He finally spoke "it's really fucking weird! You have to promise me you will never tell anyone!!" Wow. Now I'm even more curious. After swearing multiple times that I wouldn't tell anyone he says it..."I like to pie people." Wtf? What does that even mean? I ask, "like a pie pie? That you eat?" He looks very nervous, "yes a pie. Girls look so hot with pie smashed in their face. It drives me crazy!" I couldn't help but crack up laughing, it sounded so fun and silly! I wouldn't say sexy or hot, but definitely fun. "I'll do it!" I squeal enthusiastically. Once again he looks a little shocked and nervous, "Really" he asks. At this point I can see his eyes light up with complete and utter excitement. He shares with me that he's only gotten to live out this fantasy 8 times between 2 ex-girlfriends. One liked it okay, and the other didn't really care for it. This makes me sad. Sad that, for one, he was so scared of being judged for this little kink, and also sad that this turns him on so much and he's only done it 8 times at 30 years old.

For the next week I looked online to try and understand what exactly he might be looking for from me and this fetish. I wasn't sure where to look. I saw some random YouTube videos and photos but didn't really understand it. It was finally on a Friday afternoon at my neighborhood grocery that I was buying some wine and saw stacks of pies in the next cooler. Cream filled chocolate and whipped cream, lemon merengue, and a coconut meringue. I smirked and took out my phone texting the options to my pie guy. He responded almost immediately "oh wow coconut". I reply with a photo of the pie. He responds "oh dear god". I reply "it's pretty". He responds "a pretty pie for a pretty face." I'm not sure what happened but when he texts this my panties feel suddenly sticky and warm.

This pie sat for 4 days in my fridge taunting me! Both of us had a non-stop crazy weekend leading up to Mardi Gras day. Then the rain and cold got everyone a little snotty and under the weather; not very sexy. I had to protect this pie from a couple different house guests. My mother was after it at one point! I heard the plastic and tin noise and ran in screaming "no!!! That's not mine!" She thought I was insane but put the pie back on the refrigerator shelf. I needed this pie shoved in my face, and soon.

Finally the night came and I got a text he would be stopping over to play. Thank god. Curiosity was killing me!

I asked if he had anything in particular he wanted me to wear. He gave me a list of a few fantasies involving either a business suit, French maid, or naked is always good.

Business suit it is then! I had the perfect one bought for a job interview a few years ago. They said I was over dressed and I didn't get the job. Fuck em! Now I would put it to great use, and have a lot more fun than I would have had in it in that shitty job!

I was nervous and didn't know what to expect. I took a hot bubble bath, poured a glass of wine, and put on the black Calvin Klein skirt suit with a black and white zebra print blouse underneath. I then braided my hair in two long pigtail style braids, and put on a little makeup (I never wear makeup). I placed my "pretty" pie on the kitchen counter and waited.... nervously.

Finally my beautiful blue eyed man arrived. We sat, a little awkwardly, on my sofa discussing our day and what we did over the holiday. I finally said "come on! Let's do this!" The waiting was seriously killing me at this point. I just wanted to know what the hell this was all about!

He kissed me standing and walking me backwards towards my bed, the exquisite pressure of his hands on my hips. I sat on the edge of bed looking up at him. His baby face, and smirk, and those damned gorgeous blue eyes make me melt! He walked away into kitchen to retrieve my coconut present. I just stared, loving every moment of watching him and the underlying excitement that glowed from that little smile on his face. He sat the pie on the table next to my bed and his hands moved to his zipper to slide off his pants.

I sighed heavily feeling the tightness in my stomach that I always feel knowing he will soon be inside of me. I could feel my clit lightly twitching and he had barely touched me yet. He leaned over, pulled my black skirt up and placed a warm hand on my wet pussy and began rubbing me gently. I moaned contently, feeling my entire body relax in one deep breath. He then took my legs in each hand and lifted them up above his shoulders sliding inside of me gently before starting a pounding rhythm that brought me quickly to climax. I could feel my muscles tightening on his hard cock with each wave of orgasm.

When I opened my eyes he was holding the thick creamy coconut pie in his hand. Looking at the 2 inches of whipped cream I suddenly wanted to scream! I started giggling, my eyes darting back and forth between his gleaming eyes and the pie in his hand. I heard a low groan deep in his throat and he began moving inside me again. All I could concentrate on was that pie and wondering when it would be slammed into my face and what it was going to feel like. I saw a slight arm movement and flinched, then I heard that groan again. He licked his smirking lips staring at my face. Then it came! In one fast movement, I took a giant gulp of air and closed my eyes, the pie squished and squashed into my face! The cold cream was luxurious and delicious! All my senses were tingling. I felt the cold wetness dripping down my neck and him pushing the tin up my face to the top of my head. I opened my mouth again for another gulp of air smiling and giggling with delight. I couldn't see him but I could hear his breath quicken and feel a slight tremble in his legs. I felt his hot cum run between my legs and down my thigh.

I loved this. I loved only hearing and feeling him. I loved the feel, smell, and taste of the coconut pie on my skin. I loved that this was not only something I could give him, but that I wanted it too.

I put my hands to my face and wiped the pie out of my eyes. I opened them to see his beaming blue eyes smiling. He collapsed on top of me kissing me deeply again. I giggled when he pulled back and had white fluffy cream on his nose. Mmmmm! He asked if I wanted to hop in shower. I didn't, but said ok anyway. I'm finding I also am in love with cleanup. The laughter and feeling of having a dirty secret you share is beautiful. Thank god he climbed in with me, the assistance he provided pulling tiny coconut shards from my hair was greatly appreciated.

So, here I am, and that's how I got here. I hope whoever takes the time to read this enjoys it and feels free to send me a friend request, message, or mixture advice. I have a few photos from my second (french maid) wam session with blue eyes, and hopefully will have many more to come!

6

BOUND TO BE PIED

Centuries ago lawbreakers were often sentenced to displays of public humiliation, including being put in stocks in the public square. For whatever reason, sometimes the psychopath peasants would throw food and mud at the criminal in order to further humiliate them. Today? We willingly do this. One of the great things about sploshing is how easy it is to integrate it with other kinks and fetishes. Are you a top who wants to find unique ways to punish your sub? Then sploshing might be for you! (Google Mistress Shae who is a good resource for this. She goes into how various tastes, temperatures, and textures play into punishing someone with food.) Or maybe you simply want to hogtie your partner and hit them with pies. The possibilities are endless.

Foot play incorporates well with food. The sensation of sliding your toes into a bowl of batter then using your foot to paint your partner's face. Or simply have him lick them clean. Or maybe filling shoes with goo and slipping your feet inside. By adding mess you're simply adding an additional dimension with which to play.

SPLAT!

Ageplay is nothing new. There are thousands of daddy doms and littles out here watching cartoons, coloring in books, and sharing happy meals. But I wonder what a bratty little would do if she had some extra deserts in front of her. Could she pick up that whole slice of pie without her daddy noticing? Perhaps. But if he catches her, well. If she wants to play with her food, lets see how she likes it!

7

ADDITIONAL RESOURCES

The information contained in this guide was never meant to be exhaustive. There are amazing resources at your fingertips. Not just informative websites, but individuals within the community. Connecting with others and engaging in dialogue is a fantastic way to learn from others mistakes and successes. I would encourage you to visit the Ultimate Messy Directory (www.umd.net), where you will find forums filled with years of experience, stories, and sploshing videos and pictures. If you want some great inspiration, this is the place. In addition to this book the UMD is a great way to introducing sploshing to your partner. By showing them a video of something that specifically turns you on, they can have a better idea of exactly what it is you enjoy.

Messy Supplies is a UK based supplier of all things gunge. They sell colored gunge powder of all kinds. Many swear by their quality, and if you're in the UK you can get premixed gunge sent to your house, making life all the easier.

Any warehouse club is going to make shopping easy if you're planning on having any large sessions. Nobody bats an eye if you're buying a 5 pound box of cake mix. Options are limited here, but what they have they have lots of. Also, you can get free samples, so that's always a plus.

Gordon Food Service Store is an outstanding resource if you're lucky enough to have one nearby. You can find them in the Midwest, Northeast, and Florida. Here you'll find food service grade jugs of chocolate syrup, huge bags of oatmeal, frozen pies, and more. The best part is you don't have to have a membership in order to shop here, so you have nothing to lose.

8

TAKING THE PLUNGE

Do you remember your first real roller coaster? For me it was the Anaconda, at King's Dominion in Virginia. The twisted mass of metal was constructed over a pond. It dipped into a tunnel under the water and propelled you into a double look and a corkscrew. It was awe inspiring to someone who had never really done anything like that before. The Anaconda was brand new, shiny and green. And, as most go, right out of the gate you're slowly climbing that first hill. Every single click and clack built anticipation for the plunge you knew was coming. I felt pretty awesome standing in line. I was going to ride a real roller coaster; how awesome is that?

I made it a point to sit in the first row so I could see everything coming (something that stuck with me ever since). I was perfectly fine, until the harness came down over my head. Suddenly I froze. Rather than being comforted by the pressure of the safety equipment, I felt a wave of anxiety. When we started moving up the hill, I felt uncomfortable. Unsafe. There was a sense of dread. I wanted off this thing right fucking now! About halfway up it occurred to me how silly I was acting. I realized it was just a roller coaster. That people ride these things every single day and don't get hurt. A physical sense of relief came over me. By the time I got to the top of the hill I was smiling. Then screaming. And then it was over.

Diving into something new can be stressful, especially if it's something you're altogether familiar with. But sploshing isn't rocket science; you don't need to have any sort of art degree or to be a talented domme with years under your whip to try sploshing. There is zero pretentiousness about the whole thing. Because after all, who can take anyone seriously when they're covered in pie? I think that's part of the beauty of sploshing. All the stresses of the world, the bullshit we deal with every single day. And then for a couple of hours you can engage in something so equally sensual and silly without any repercussions whatsoever. How amazing is that?

This book was never intended to be an exhaustive accounting of sploshing. In reality it's so subjective and individualistic it's really impossible to fully nail down. Because of that I encourage you to take a step. For you that might mean telling your significant other (which might include sharing this book). Or it might mean heading to the grocery store to prepare for a fun-filled evening. Or perhaps it's just getting on the internet and learning more about this whole wet and messy thing you've been reading about. I hope whatever you choose brings you much happiness.

ABOUT THE AUTHOR

Wamlanta has finally written a book but cannot tell his family or friends about it. How tragic is that?

He is a splosher, wannabe writer, and is in the process of reinventing his life. Other than that there isn't much to say. You can reach him on either the UMD forums or Fetlife.

Made in the USA
Columbia, SC
15 June 2025